Fast Diet Cookbook

5:2 Intermittent Fast Diet Recipes and Meal Plans For Healthy Weight Loss and Vibrant Living

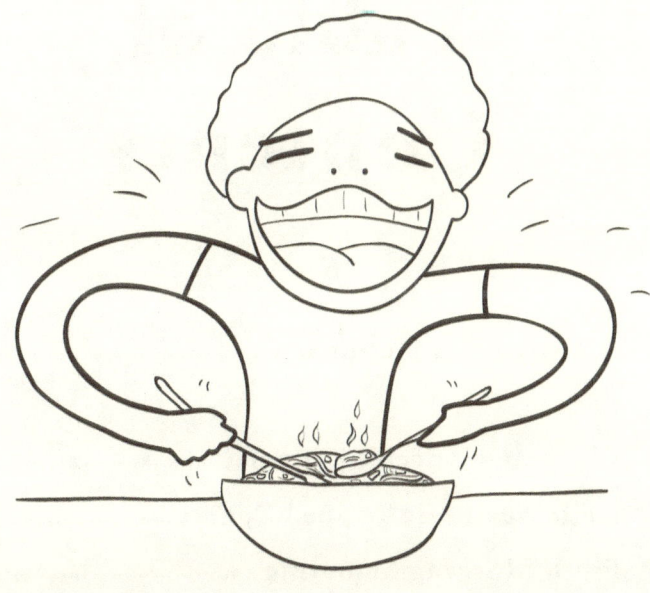

Printed in the United States of America.
First Printing, 2013

Table of Contents

A Final Word of Encouragment!

A Swift Introduction

First of all, let's give thanks.

Thank God for the fast diet!

So many so called lose weight solutions are more like a math's degree – counting calories, adding up points and sticking rigorously to a meal plan that works great so long as you don't live in the real world! Lol.

Yep, we've tried them all, and that's why the Fast diet was an epiphany for me. Not only does it allow me to eat and enjoy many of the foods I truly love, over time it has actually changed my tastes to prefer foods that my body craves, rather than just my taste buds.

Diets are a popular fad everywhere in the world and some work while others do not seem to work as well. The 5:2 diet is a diet where you eat whatever you want for 5 days of the week and then fast for 2 days of the week. The fasting takes place on two non-consecutive days.

Even though it is referred to as fasting, you still eat just a lower amount of calories. The goal is to stay under 500 calories for the entire day. You can break up the diet however you want on these fasting days by saving up for a large dinner or splitting up your meals between breakfast and dinner, lunch and dinner, or even breakfast and lunch. You will need to find what works for your body and then go with that.

The 5:2 diet has helped many people lose weight and there are many advocates of the diet. One of the coolest benefits of this diet is that you do get to eat what you want for 5 days of the week. This makes it easier on people who have a hard time sticking to a diet because it places too many restrictions or just becomes plain complicated (yours truly! ☺).

Another benefit is that you will actually shed fat and lose weight at the same time. You will eventually begin to rethink the foods that you eat as well and develop better eating habits.

Lastly, the diet also has the advantage of being flexible. You can customize the days you want to fast and the days you want to eat normally.

And it gets even better. Even while in the fasting mode, you can still enjoy delicious meals. It's true.

This book introduces you to healthy meal options that can be chosen on your fasting days. All of the meals in this book range from breakfast to dinner and all weigh-in under 500 calories.

Rather than bog you down with 20,568 recipes, we have chosen just 52 of our easiest and most delicious 5:2 recipes to share with you. Mix'n'match them for varied and satisfying meal plans for your fasting days, and watch the pounds and ounces drop away.

We have kept things easy, simple to read and put into practice. We hope you enjoy each and every one of these wonderful recipes just as much as we do.

Why wait a moment longer?

Lose weight fast with the fast diet, and still enjoy great grub even on your fasting days. It's a win-win!

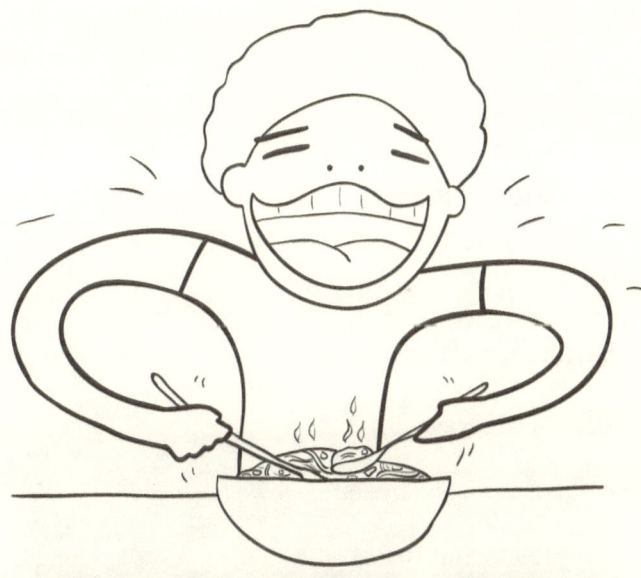

BREAKFAST

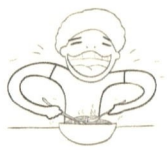

Chive and Zucchini Omelet

This omelet is the perfect size and also very delicious. Under 200 calories, this is the perfect protein packed breakfast to start your day of right.

Ingredients:

- 2 large eggs

- 1 teaspoon olive oil

- 1 zucchini, grated

- 1 teaspoon chives, minced

Directions:

1. Crack the eggs in a bowl and scramble them.

2. Add in the zucchini and mix well.

3. Season with the chives, stir.

4.   Place the olive oil in a skillet over medium high heat.

5.   Once the oil is hot, add in the egg mixture.

6.   Cook for 2 minutes on each side or until egg is set.

7.   Serve.

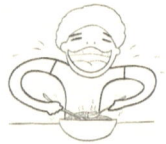

Delicious Fruit Topped Yogurt

This delicious breakfast is under 200 calories and is perfect for any morning on the go. You can whip this up easily with little effort and enjoy the delicious taste.

Ingredients:

- 1 ½ ounces sunflower seeds

- ½ apple, grated

- 5 ½ ounces yogurt, plain

- 10 blueberries, sliced

Directions:

1. Place the yogurt in a small bowl.

2. Add in the blueberries and apples, stir.

3.   Top with sunflower seeds.

4.   Serve with a smile.

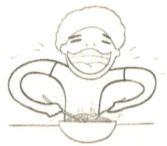

Fresh Morning Smoothie

This morning smoothie is perfect for any fast day. It is under 200 calories and sweetly flavored with fresh strawberries and banana. You will love whipping up this quick and easy smoothie any fast day of the week.

Ingredients:

- ½ cup orange juice

- ¼ cup cucumber, peeled and diced

- ¼ cup banana, peeled and sliced

- 1 lime, juiced

- 1/8 cup oats

- ¾ cup strawberries, sliced

Directions:

1. Place all of the ingredients into a blender.

2. Blend on high for 1 minute or until the mixture is completely smooth.

3. Pour into a glass and serve.

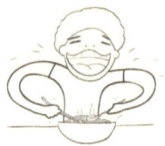

Delicious Apple and Spice Bread

This apple and spice bread is under 50 calories per serving. The bread is moist and deliciously flavored making it a great breakfast choice.

Ingredients:

- ¼ cup egg substitute

- 2 tablespoons light brown sugar

- 1 cup apple, shredded

- 1 ½ cups flour

- ½ teaspoon baking soda

- ½ teaspoon cinnamon

- ¼ teaspoon cardamom

- ½ teaspoon salt

- ¼ teaspoon nutmeg

- 1/4cup sour cream

- 2 teaspoons baking powder

Directions:

1.   Start by preheating your oven to 350 degrees.
     Grab a loaf pan and grease it with cooking spray.
     Set to the side.

2.   In a large mixing bowl, mix together the sour
     cream, apple, and egg substitute. Stir until well
     blended.

3.   Add in the remaining ingredients and stir until
     well mixed.

4.   Pour the bread batter into the loaf pan and place
     in the oven.

5.   Bake for 40 minutes or until golden brown on
     top.

6.   Remove from the oven and allow to cool slightly.

7.   Slice and serve.

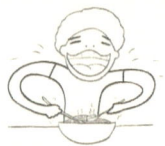

Morning Breakfast Casserole

This morning breakfast casserole is under 200 calories per serving and is a great way to eat breakfast. This breakfast casserole is both satisfying and delicious.

Ingredients:

- 1 green pepper, diced

- 4 large eggs

- 6 bacon strips

- 1 onion, diced

- 1 cup shredded cheddar cheese, reduced fat

- ½ teaspoon pepper

- ¾ teaspoon salt

- 1 cup milk, fat free

- 4 cups shredded hash browns, room temperature

- 16 ounces egg substitute

Directions:

1. Preheat your oven to 350 degrees and grease a 13 inch by 9 inch glass baking dish with cooking spray. Set aside.

2. Heat a skillet over medium heat and cook the bacon until crispy.

3. Remove the bacon from the skillet and allow to drain on paper towels. Once the bacon has cooled and drained, crumble.

4. Using the skillet with the bacon grease, warm until hot.

5. Add in the green pepper and onion.

6. Sauté in the bacon grease for 5 minutes or until tender.

7. In a large mixing bowl, whisk together the eggs and egg substitute. Add in the milk and whisk until mixed.

8.   Stir in the cheese, hashbrowns, bacon, onion, green pepper, salt and pepper. Stir well until completely mixed.

9.   Pour the mixture into the greased baking dish and place in the oven.

10.   Bake for 35 minutes or until the eggs are set and the center is cooked throughout.

11.   Serve.

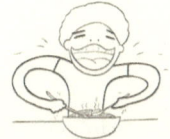

Nutty Granola

This granola recipe is more flavorful than traditional granola and also very filling. Under 130 calories for ¼ cup makes this recipe perfect for a morning treat. You can eat this granola alone or simply add it to some plain yogurt.

Ingredients:

- ½ cup shredded coconut

- ¼ cup oat bran

- 2 cups oats

- ½ cup wheat germ

- ¼ cup almonds, slivered

- ¼ cup sunflower kernels

- 2 tablespoons sesame seeds

- ¼ cup pecans, chopped

- 2 tablespoons olive oil

- ¼ cup honey

- 2 tablespoon orange peel, grated

- ½ teaspoon salt

- 1 teaspoon vanilla extract

- 1 cup cranberries, dried

- 3 tablespoons raisins

- ½ cup figs, dried

- ¾ cup dates, chopped

- ½ cup apricots, dried and chopped

Directions:

1. Preheat the oven for 350 degrees.

2. In a large mixing bowl, mix together the coconut, oats, wheat germ, sunflower kernels, oat bran, pecans, almonds, and sesame seeds.

3.   In a separate small mixing bowl, whisk together
        the vanilla, honey, orange peel, oil, and salt
        together until well combined.

4.   Pour the honey mixture over the oat mixture and
        toss until well coated.

5.   Pour the oat mixture onto an ungreased baking
        sheet and place in the oven for 25 minutes,
        stirring half way through cooking.

6.   Remove from the oven and allow to cool.

7.   Stir in the dates, cranberries, raisins, apricots, and
        figs.

8.   Serve.

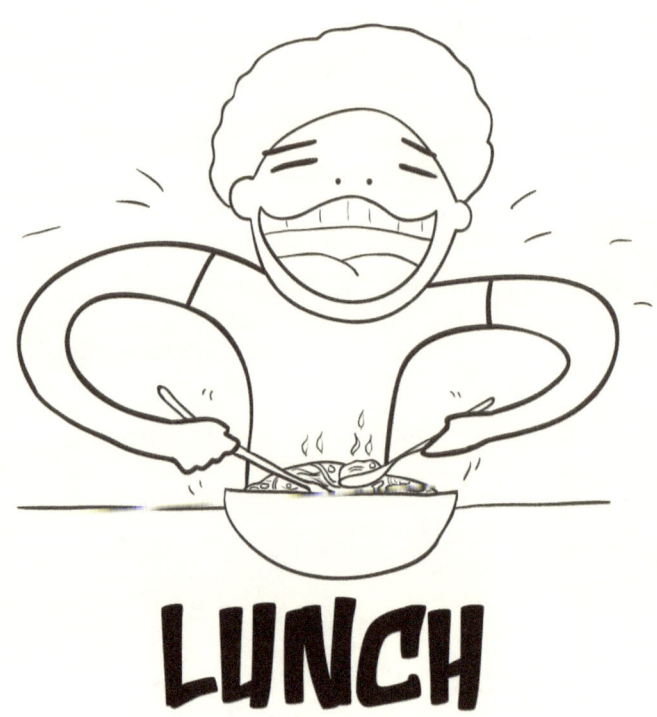

LUNCH

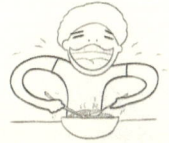

Delicious Bean Salad

This is a great and healthy lunch recipe to help you power through your day. The beans in this recipe are deliciously dressed and served with cheese for the perfect combination.

Ingredients:

- 1 teaspoon mustard

- 2 tablespoons olive oil

- 1 tablespoon white wine vinegar

- 2 tablespoons mint leaves

- ½ cup soya beans, frozen

- ½ cup sugar snap peas, trimmed

- ½ cup green beans, trimmed

- ¾ cup feta cheese, crumbled

- ½ cup baby beetroot, sliced

Directions:

1. Place the olive oil, vinegar and mustard in a small bowl. Whisk together until mixed well. Set to the side.

2. Place a pot of water on the stove over high heat and allow to come to a boil.

3. Once the water is boiling, add salt.

4. Add the soya beans to the boiling water and cook for 3 minutes. Add in the snap peas and green beans. Continue to boil for another 2 minutes.

5. Drain the beans from the water and allow them to sit under cold water until cooled down.

6. Place the beans in a large mixing bowl.

7. Stir in the mint leaves, beetroot and feta cheese until well mixed.

8. Pour the dressing over top of the green bean mixture and toss well.

9. Serve.

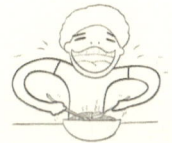

Portobello Quesadilla

This is a hearty and perfect lunch time meal that is under 300 calories for both quesadilla pockets. You will enjoy the meaty taste of the Portobello with the crunchy vegetables.

Ingredients:

- 1 lime, juiced

- ¼ cup water

- 1 tablespoon Italian seasoning

- 2 tablespoons canola oil

- ¼ teaspoon salt

- ¼ teaspoon pepper

- 1 teaspoon garlic, minced

- ¼ teaspoon ground cumin

23

- 1/8 teaspoon cayenne pepper

- 1 red onion, sliced

- 1 yellow bell pepper, sliced

- 1 red bell pepper, sliced

- 1 zucchini, sliced into ¼ inch slices

- 1 pound baby Portobello mushrooms

- 1 cup shredded cheddar cheese, reduced-fat

- 8 slices pita bread, cut in half

Directions:

1. In a large mixing bowl, combine the lime juice, water, Italian seasoning, canola oil, garlic, cumin, salt, pepper, and cayenne. Stir until mixed well.

2. Place the onion, zucchini, mushrooms, and peppers in the sauce mixture and coat well.

3. Cover and refrigerate overnight.

4. The next day, remove the bowl from the refrigerator and remove the vegetables from the marinade.

5.   Heat a skillet over medium high heat and coat with cooking spray.

6.   Once hot, add the vegetables to the skillet and cook for 10 minutes or until the vegetables are tender but still crisp.

7.   Sprinkle the cheese on top of the vegetables and continue cooking for an additional 2 minutes.

8.   Place ½ cup of the vegetable mixture into each of the pita halves.

9.   Serve.

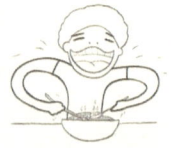

Cheesy Eggplant

This is a great lunch recipe under 120 calories. The eggplant is tender and provides enough protein to get you through the rest of your day.

Ingredients:

- 1 can (14 ½ ounces) stewed tomatoes

- 1 ½ pounds eggplant

- 2 teaspoons sugar

- ½ teaspoon salt

- 1 teaspoon flour

- ½ teaspoon paprika

- ½ teaspoon garlic powder

- ¼ teaspoon pepper

- ¼ teaspoon dried oregano

- 2 tablespoons parmesan cheese

- 2/3 cup shredded mozzarella cheese, reduced fat

Directions:

1. Preheat your oven to 350 degrees and lightly grease a 13 inch by 9 inch baking dish with cooking spray.

2. Grab the eggplant and slice it into slices that are about a ½ inch thick.

3. Place the eggplant slices into a saucepan and cover them with water.

4. Place the saucepan over high heat and allow to boil.

5. Once the water boils, reduce heat, cover, and simmer for 5 minutes.

6. Drain the eggplants and dry.

7. In a separate saucepan, mix together the tomatoes, flour, sugar, salt, pepper, garlic powder, oregano, and paprika.

8. Allow to heat over medium heat for 5 minutes or until thickened.

9. Layer the eggplant in the greased baking dish and top with the tomato sauce.

10.   Sprinkle with the cheese and cover.

11.   Bake for 20 minutes and then uncover and continue baking for another 10 minutes.

12.   Remove and allow to cool slightly.

13.   Serve.

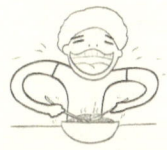

Potato Wedges with Parmesan

Ingredients:

- 1 teaspoon olive oil

- 1 large potato, cut into wedges about ¼ inch thick

- 2 cups water, cold

- 1 tablespoon parmesan cheese

- 1/8 teaspoon salt

- 1/8 teaspoon pepper

- 1/8 teaspoon sage

Directions:

1. Place the water and potatoes in a saucepan and allow to heat to boiling over high heat.

2. Boil the potatoes for 5 minutes or until tender but crisp.

3. Remove the potatoes from the saucepan and rinse under cold water. Dry.

4. Place oil in a skillet over medium high heat.

5. Once the oil is hot, add in the potatoes and cook them for 5-10 minutes or until browned.

6. Season with salt, pepper, sage, and parmesan cheese.

7. Serve.

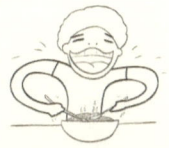

Tuna Wrap
with Sundried Tomatoes

This tuna wrap is the perfect size for lunch and is under 300 calories. You will enjoy the tomatoes mixed in as they add a nice flavor to the tuna.

Ingredients:

- ¼ cup sundried tomatoes, minced

- 12 ounces chunk light tuna in water, drained and flaked

- 2 tablespoons parsley, chopped

- 3 tablespoons mayonnaise, low fat

- 2 tablespoons Dijon mustard

- 4 leaves green leaf lettuce

- 4 (8-inch) whole wheat tortillas

Directions:

1. In a small bowl, mix together the tomatoes, tuna, parsley, mayonnaise and pepper. Mix well to combine all ingredients.

2. Spread ½ teaspoon of mustard onto each of the tortillas.

3. Top each tortilla with a lettuce leaf.

4. Evenly spread the tuna mixture on top of each lettuce leaf and then roll up the tortilla into a wrap.

5. Serve.

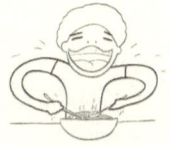

Fresh Grilled Cheese

This is a grown up version of grilled cheese and is perfect for anyone. This lunch favorite only has 230 calories.

Ingredients:

- 1 1/3 cups roasted red bell peppers, sliced

- 8 slices whole wheat bread

- 8 teaspoons Dijon mustard

- ½ cup artichoke hearts, drained and sliced

- 1 cup shredded cheddar cheese, reduced fat

Directions:

1. Spread the Dijon mustard evenly on the slices of bread (1 tsp. of mustard per slice).

2.   Top 4 of the slices of bread with the cheese.

3.   Place 2 tablespoons of the artichoke hearts on top of the cheese and 1/3 cup of the peppers on top of the artichoke hearts.

4.   Top with a slice of bread to make a sandwich.

5.   Spray cooking spray in a skillet and allow to heat over medium heat.

6.   Once hot, add the sandwiches and allow to cook for 2 minutes on each side or until golden brown.

7.   Slice and serve.

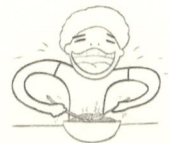

Potato Salad

Many people only get to enjoy potato salad at a barbecue or cook out. This recipe is quick and easy to make. Did we mention it only has 85 calories per serving? Enjoy this for lunch any day of the week.

Ingredients:

- 1 ½ cups celery, sliced

- 2/3 cup light mayonnaise

- 24 ounces frozen diced hashbrown potatoes with peppers and onions

- 1 tablespoon mustard

- 1 tablespoon sugar

- 8 ounces light sour cream

- ½ teaspoon salt

- 1 tablespoon white wine vinegar

- 3 hard boil eggs, chopped

Directions:

1. Place the hashbrown in a large saucepan and cover with water. Bring to a boil over high heat.

2. Cook hashbrowns for 8 minutes or until tender. Drain.

3. In a large mixing bowl, toss the hashbrowns and celery together.

4. In a small mixing bowl, whisk together the mayonnaise, sour cream, mustard, sugar, vinegar, and salt.

5. Add the mayonnaise mixture to the hashbrowns and stir to coat evenly and well.

6. Fold in the eggs.

7. Cover and allow to chill in the refrigerator.

8. Serve.

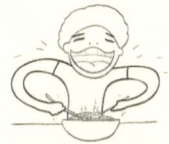

Spicy Chicken Salad

Ingredients:

- 4 boneless, skinless chicken breast halves

- 3 tablespoons jerk marinade

- ¼ teaspoon salt

- 1 orange, juiced

- 2 tablespoons honey

- 2 mangoes, peeled and sliced

- 1 red onion, sliced

- 2 tablespoons balsamic vinegar

- 2 teaspoons olive oil

Directions:

1.   In a large mixing bowl, pour the jerk marinade
        over top of the chicken. Coat the chicken evenly
        on both sides.

2.   Cover the bowl and allow the chicken to marinate
        in the refrigerator for 1 hour.

3.   Heat the oven to broil.

4.   Remove the chicken from the refrigerator and
        place on a greased baking sheet.

5.   Cook the chicken in the oven for 10-15 minutes
        or until cooked throughout.

6.   Remove from the oven and allow to cool while
        making the sauce.

7.   In a mixing bowl, whisk together the honey,
        balsamic vinegar, olive oil, salt, mangoes, orange
        juice, and onion.

8.   Pour the sauce over the chicken and coat evenly.

9.   Place lettuce leaves on a serving plate and evenly
        place the chicken on top of each lettuce leaf.

10.   Serve.

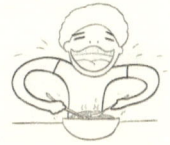

Colorful Turkey Salad

Who said you can only have turkey during the fall season? This turkey salad is delicious and also colorful. It makes a great lunch time meal and will satisfy; all under 100 calories.

Ingredients:

- 1 ½ cups peas, frozen

- 1 ½ pounds turkey breast, cooked and cubed

- ¼ cup red bell pepper, chopped

- ¼ cup yellow bell pepper, chopped

- ½ cup celery, chopped

- ½ cup carrots, chopped

- ¼ cup scallions, chopped

- ½ teaspoon pepper

- ¼ teaspoon salt

- 1 teaspoon onion powder

- 1 teaspoon garlic powder

- 1 cup light mayonnaise

Directions:

1. In a large mixing bowl, toss the peas, pepper, carrot, turkey, celery and scallion until well combined.

2. Grab a small mixing bowl and whisk together the mayonnaise, salt, pepper, garlic powder, and onion powder.

3. Pour the dressing over the turkey mixture and toss well.

4. Cover and allow to chill in the refrigerator for a few hours.

5. Serve.

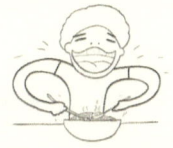

Shrimp and Cucumber Sandwich

This is a refreshing sandwich that will power you throughout the rest of your day. The cucumbers and shrimp pair nicely together with the cream cheese and seasonings. This sandwich is less than 300 calories.

Ingredients:

- 6 small French bread rolls

- 1/3 cup scallions, minced

- ¼ cup light mayonnaise

- ¼ cup low fat cream cheese, softened

- ½ teaspoon garlic salt

- ¼ cup yogurt, low fat and plain

- ¼ teaspoon pepper

- 1 cup cucumbers, sliced thin

- 1 ½ pounds shrimp, cooked, peeled and deveined

- 6 leaves lettuce

- ½ cup radishes, sliced thin

Directions:

1. In a large mixing bowl, combine the cream cheese, scallions, yogurt, mayonnaise, pepper and garlic salt. Mix well.

2. Cut the French read rolls in half lengthwise to open them up.

3. Spread the cream cheese mixture evenly over the rolls.

4. Place the shrimp evenly on top of the cream cheese spread on the rolls.

5. Place the cucumber on top of the shrimp and then top with lettuce and radishes.

6. Serve.

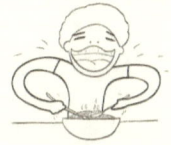

Vegetable and Steak Salad

This is a great lunch item that you will want to add to your weekly menu. This salad comes in under 300 calories and is also very delicious.

Ingredients:

- 1 zucchini, diced

- 1 red bell pepper, sliced

- 1 yellow bell pepper, sliced

- 1 green pepper, sliced

- 1 pound beef tenderloin steaks, cut into 1 inch cubes

- 1 baby eggplant, diced

- 16 small mushrooms

- 1 onion, cut into 1 inch wedges

- 8 cups salad greens, chopped

- ¼ teaspoon salt

- ¾ cup Italian salad dressing, non-fat

- 2 tablespoons balsamic vinegar

- 1 teaspoon dried oregano

- ¼ teaspoon pepper

- 2 garlic cloves, minced

Directions:

1. Preheat your oven to 425 degrees and grease a jellyroll pan with cooking spray.

2. Place all of the vegetables in the greased pan.

3. In a small bowl, combine the garlic, balsamic vinegar, pepper, and oregano. Whisk together until mixed.

4. Pour this mixture over the vegetables and place in the oven.

5. Bake for 35 minutes or until the vegetables are tender.

6.   In a large skillet over medium high heat cook the beef steaks for 15 minutes or until cooked to desired doneness.

7.   Once the steaks are done cooking, remove from the skillet and allow to rest.

8.   Season the steak with the salt and then slice crosswise.

9.   Place salad greens evenly on plates and top with vegetables.

10. Place steaks on top of vegetables and then drizzle with salad dressing.

11. Serve.

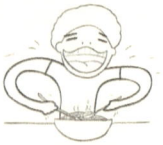

Coleslaw

Coleslaw is a favorite among many people and is often served at barbecues and also entertaining events. This recipe is perfect for lunch whenever you are craving coleslaw and is less than 65 calories per serving.

Ingredients:

- 2 tablespoons apple cider vinegar

- 1 cup light sour cream

- ½ teaspoon salt

- 1 tablespoon sugar

- ½ teaspoon pepper

- 2 ½ cups green cabbage, sliced thin

- 2 ½ cups red cabbage, sliced thin

- 1 yellow squash, cut into strips

- 1 zucchini, cut into strips

- 3 carrots, shredded

- ¼ cup parsley, chopped

Directions:

1. In a large mixing bowl, whisk together the vinegar, sour cream, salt, sugar, and pepper. Make sure this mixture is combined well.

2. Add in the vegetables and stir well to coat with mayonnaise mixture.

3. Fold in the parsley.

4. Serve.

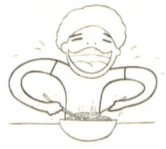

Pear Salad with Bleu Cheese

This salad is under 110 calories and is perfect for a cheese and fruit delight. This salad is perfect for lunch and can be enjoyed whenever you want.

Ingredients:

- 2 slices turkey bacon, cooked and crumbled

- 8 ounces salad greens

- 1 lemon, juiced

- 2 tablespoons walnuts, chopped

- 1 pear, cored and chopped

- 1/3 cup bleu cheese dressing

Directions:

1.   Place the lemon juice in a small bowl and add in the pear. Toss to coat the pears evenly. Drain.

2.   Place the pears in a large bowl and add in the walnuts, dressing, bacon, and salad greens. Toss well until completely coated.

3.   Serve.

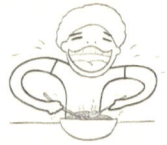

Delicious Au Gratin

This Au Gratin is made with Spinach and cheese making it extra tasty and delightful. Each serving is under 120 calories. Fill up on this lunch recipe.

Ingredients:

- ¼ cup cream cheese, fat free and cubed

- 2 (10 ounce) packages spinach, frozen and chopped

- ¼ cup feta cheese, crumbled

- ½ cup egg substitute

- ½ cup skim milk

- 2 tablespoons scallions, sliced

- ½ cup water chestnuts, chopped

- ¾ cup breadcrumbs

- ¼ teaspoon garlic salt

- 2 teaspoons butter, melted

- 1 tablespoon parmesan cheese

Directions:

1. Cook the spinach in a saucepan according to the directions on the package. Drain and squeeze out as much moisture as possible.

2. Place the spinach back in the saucepan.

3. Add the feta and cream cheese to the saucepan and stir until the cream cheese is melted.

4. Add in the egg substitute, milk, scallions, garlic salt, and water chestnuts. Mix well.

5. Grab a 2 quart casserole dish and spray with cooking spray.

6. Place the spinach mixture in the casserole dish.

7. Preheat the oven to 350 degrees.

8. Place the breadcrumbs, butter, and parmesan cheese in a small bowl. Mix together well.

9. Sprinkle the breadcrumbs over the spinach.

10. Place in the oven and bake for 45 minutes or until set and the breadcrumbs are golden brown.

11. Serve.

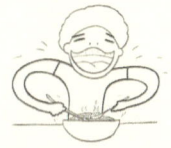

Fresh Red Beans and Rice

This is a great Spanish dish for lunch. This recipe is under 150 calories and will help keep you full until dinner time.

Ingredients:

- 1 onion, chopped

- 1 red bell pepper, chopped

- 1 teaspoon olive oil

- 1 tablespoon thyme, chopped

- 2 ¼ cups water

- 1 teaspoon minced garlic

- 1 (15 ounce) can red kidney beans, rinsed and drained

- 1 cup long grain rice

- ½ teaspoon salt

- ½ teaspoon cayenne pepper

Directions:

1.   Place the oil in a skillet and allow to heat over medium high heat.

2.   Once the oil is hot, add in the garlic, red pepper, and onion.

3.   Cook for 5 minutes or until tender.

4.   Add in the salt, thyme, rice, cayenne, and water.

5.   Allow the mixture to come to a boil.

6.   Reduce the heat and cover the pot.

7.   Simmer for 20 minutes or until the rice is tender.

8.   Add in the beans and remove the pan from the heat.

9.   Cover and allow the beans to stand for 5 minutes.

10.   Remove the lid and stir.

11.   Serve.

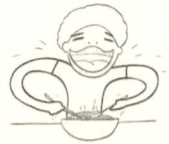

Pasta Salad

This pasta salad is easy to make and also very delicious. It is the perfecto combination of meat, noodles, and vegetables. This lunch recipe is under 215 calories.

Ingredients:

- 1 tablespoon mustard

- 6 pickles, chopped

- 1 cup rotini pasta

- 4 tablespoons reduced fat Italian dressing

- 3 tablespoons parsley, chopped

- 8 slices pastrami

- 18 cherry tomatoes, halved

Directions:

1.   Cook the pasta according to the package directions.

2.   In a mixing bowl, whisk together the mustard and Italian dressing until combined.

3.   Add in the pickles, pastrami, tomatoes, and parsley. Toss well.

4.   Drain the pasta.

5.   Pour the dressing and vegetable mix over the pasta and toss well to evenly coat.

6.   Serve.

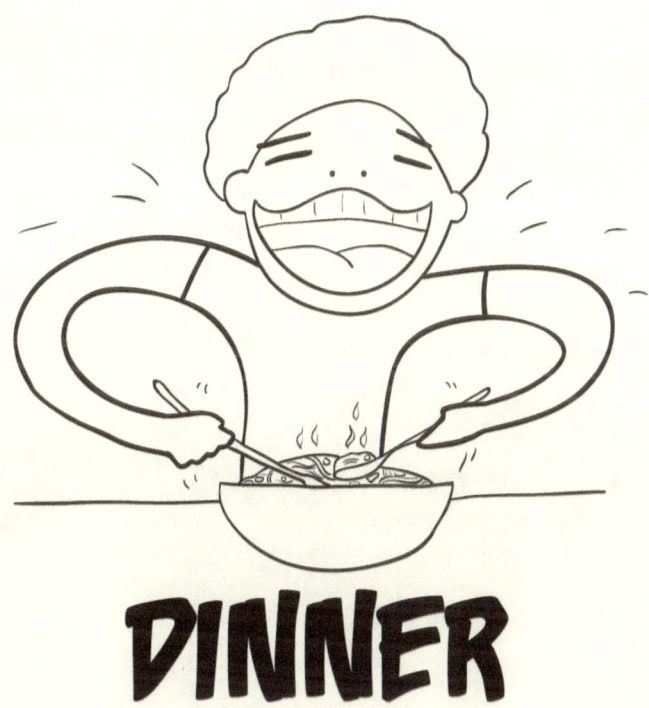

DINNER

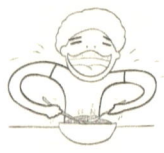

Skewered Pork

This is the perfect dinner dish that will keep you pleased and is very delicious. This dish is 200 calories and will definitely be a family favorite.

Ingredients:

- ½ teaspoon ground ginger

- 2 tablespoons parsley, chopped

- 1 teaspoon ground coriander

- 3 tablespoons olive oil

- ¼ teaspoon pepper

- ¼ teaspoon salt

- 2 garlic cloves, minced

- 1 ½ pounds pork fillet, cut into bite sized pieces

- 1 lemon, zested and juiced

- 18 mini skewers

Directions:

1. In a large mixing bowl, whisk together the garlic, lemon juice, lemon zest, parsley, ginger and coriander.

2. Season the pork with salt and pepper.

3. Place the pork in the marinade and coat evenly.

4. Take the skewers and thread 3 pieces of pork onto each skewer.

5. Preheat your grill.

6. Once the grill is preheated, place the pork on the grill and allow to cook for 10 minutes or until cooked through.

7. Remove the skewers from the grill and serve.

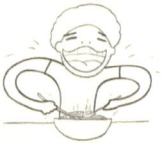

Cashew, Vegetable, and Chicken Stir Fry

This delicious stir fry is the perfect combination of cashews, chicken and vegetables. This recipe is perfect for dinner and under 260 calories.

Ingredients:

- 1 tablespoon olive oil

- ¼ cup cashews, chopped

- 1 yellow bell pepper, chopped

- 1 red onion, sliced

- 1 pound boneless, skinless chicken breast fillets, cut into 1 inch pieces

- 1 garlic clove, minced

- 3 tablespoons soy sauce

- ¾ cup broccoli, chopped

- 2 tablespoons sweet chili sauce

Directions:

1. Heat skillet over medium high heat and cook the cashew nuts for 30 seconds.

2. Remove the cashew nuts and then add oil to the skillet.

3. Once the oil is hot, add in the onion and pepper. Cook for 5 minutes or until tender.

4. Add in the chicken and continue to cook for 3 minutes or until the chicken is cooked through.

5. Stir in the broccoli and garlic and cook for 2 minutes.

6. Drizzle the chili sauce and soy sauce over top of the mixture and stir. Continue to cook for another 2 minutes.

7. Sprinkle with cashews and serve.

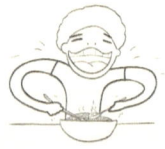

Hearty Beef Stew

Beef stew is a very warm and inviting meal. You can enjoy this delicious dinner whenever you want and it is all under 250 calories per serving.

Ingredients:

- 1 red onion, chopped

- 1 pound stewing beef

- 2 garlic cloves, minced

- 2 cups beef stock

- 1 1/3 cups baby carrots

- 2 tablespoons balsamic vinegar

- 2 tablespoons sun-dried tomato paste

- 2 tablespoons gravy granules

Directions:

1. Preheat your oven to 350 degrees and grease a casserole dish.

2. Place the beef, garlic, onion, beef stock, carrots, vinegar, tomato paste, and gravy granules in the casserole dish.

3. Stir well to combine.

4. Cook in the oven for 90 minutes or until the meat is cooked through and the vegetables are tender.

5. Serve.

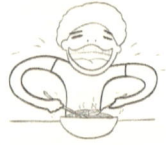

Chicken Tikka Masala

This 200 calorie recipe is a great dinner dish and will keep you satisfied. This dish is packed with a ton of flavor and easy to make.

Ingredients:

- 1 ½ pounds boneless, skinless chicken breast fillets

- 1 tablespoon olive oil

- 6 tablespoons tikka masala paste

- 1 can (14-16 ounces) tomatoes, chopped

- ½ cup water

- 1 red onion, sliced

Directions:

1.   Place the oil in a skillet and heat over medium high heat.

2.   Cook the onion for 5 minutes or until tender.

3.   Add in the chicken and cook for 10 minutes or until cooked through.

4.   Slowly stir in the tikka masala paste and mix well to combine. Allow to cook for 5 minutes.

5.   Add in tomatoes and also water. Stir to mix.

6.   Allow to warm in the skillet for 5 minutes and then serve.

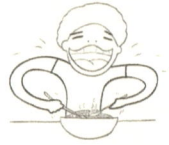

Spinach Lasagna Rolls

These lasagna rolls are very tasty and instead of meat use spinach. They are great for you and only carry 240 calories per serving.

Ingredients:

- 1 tablespoon olive oil

- 10 whole wheat lasagna noodles, cooked and drained

- 2 garlic cloves, minced

- 24 ounces spaghetti sauce

- 1 cup low fat ricotta cheese

- ½ cup low fat cottage cheese

- 1 ½ cups shredded mozzarella cheese, reduced fat

- 6 cups baby spinach, chopped

- 1 large egg white

- ¼ teaspoon salt

- 1 teaspoon dried oregano

- ¼ cup parmesan cheese

- ½ teaspoon pepper

Directions:

1. Preheat your oven to 425 degrees and grease a 13 inch by 9 inch casserole dish. Set aside.

2. In a skillet over medium high heat, allow oil to warm.

3. Once the oil is hot, cook the garlic for 1 minute.

4. Add in the spinach and continue to cook for an additional 4 minutes.

5. In a mixing bowl, mix together the cottage cheese, 1 cup mozzarella cheese, spinach and garlic mixture, ricotta cheese, egg white, salt, pepper and oregano.

6. Place the lasagna noodles on a flat surface and add ¼ cup of the cheese mixture to each noodle. Spread over the noodles to coat them evenly.

7. Roll the noodle up into a roll formation and place seam side down in the casserole dish.

8. Spread the pasta sauce over top of the noodles and sprinkle with remaining mozzarella cheese.

9. Sprinkle with parmesan cheese and cover.

10. Bake in the oven for 20 minutes or until cheese is melted.

11. Serve.

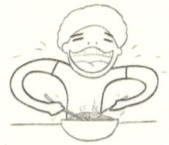

Roasted Vegetables with Sausage

This is a great under 275 calorie dinner for any day of the week. The vegetables are perfectly roasted until tender.

Ingredients:

- 2 garlic cloves, minced

- 12 sausages

- 1 zucchini, diced

- 2 red onions, cut into wedges

- 2 yellow bell peppers, chopped

- 18 cherry tomatoes, halved

- 2 tablespoons olive oil

Directions:

1. Preheat your oven to 375 degrees and grease a baking dish.

2. Place the sausage in the baking dish and allow to cook for 5 minutes in the oven.

3. Remove from the oven and add in the garlic, onion, pepper and zucchini.

4. Drizzle the vegetables with oil.

5. Allow to cook in the oven for 25 minutes and then remove from the oven.

6. Turn the sausage and vegetables over and add in the tomatoes.

7. Return to the oven and continue roasting for 5 more minutes.

8. Serve.

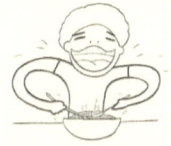

Stuffed Peppers

These stuffed peppers are seasoned to perfection with Italian flavors. At 165 calories, these peppers are the perfect dinner portion.

Ingredients:

- 1 red onion, sliced

- 2 teaspoons olive oil

- 4 ounces mushrooms, chopped

- 1 zucchini, diced

- 1 (14 ounce) can tomatoes, diced

- 1 garlic clove, minced

- 1 ounce pine nuts

- 1 tablespoon tomato paste

- ¼ cup parmesan cheese

- 4 yellow bell peppers, tops and seeds removed

- 2 tablespoon basil, chopped

- ¼ teaspoon salt

- ¼ teaspoon pepper

Directions:

1. Preheat your oven to 350 degrees and grease a casserole dish with cooking spray. Set aside.

2. Heat a skillet over medium high heat and add the oil.

3. Once the oil is hot, add in the onion, mushrooms, zucchini, and garlic. Cook for 5 minutes or until the vegetables are tender.

4. Slowly stir in the tomato paste and canned tomatoes.

5. Allow the mixture to come to a boil and then reduce the heat.

6. Simmer for 15 minutes or until the sauce starts to thicken.

7. Remove the pan from the heat and stir in the basil,

salt, pepper, and pine nuts.

8.   Slice the peppers in half lengthwise.

9.   Place the peppers in a saucepan and cover with water.

10.   Allow the water to boil for 3 minutes and then drain.

11.   Put the peppers, cut side up, in the casserole dish.

12.   Evenly spread the vegetable stuffing mixture over the pepper halves. Cover the pan with foil and place in the oven.

13.   Bake for 20 minutes. Remove from the oven and uncover.

14.   Sprinkle the peppers with the parmesan cheese and return to the oven for another 10 minutes.

15.   Remove from the oven and serve.

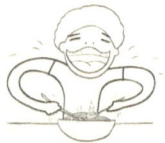

Broccoli and Shrimp Scampi

This recipe is only 185 calories and is sure to please. You can whip this up easily and you don't even need to go to a restaurant to get shrimp that tastes this good.

Ingredients:

- 1 tablespoon minced garlic

- 1 tablespoon olive oil

- 1 pound large shrimp, peeled and deveined

- ½ teaspoon crushed red pepper

- 2/3 cup water

- ½ teaspoon cornstarch

- 4 cups broccoli florets

- 2 tablespoons basil, chopped

- 2/3 cup clam juice

- 1 lemon, juiced

- ¼ teaspoon salt

- ¼ teaspoon pepper

Directions:

1. Heat a large skillet over medium heat.

2. Place ½ tablespoon of the oil in the skillet and allow to warm.

3. Once the oil is hot, add in ½ tablespoon of the garlic and the red pepper. Stir well and allow to cook for 1 minute.

4. Add in the shrimp and season with the salt.

5. Cook the shrimp until they are pink, about 4 minutes.

6. Remove the shrimp mixture from the skillet and place in a bowl. Set aside.

7. Add the remaining olive oil to the skillet and allow to heat.

8. Once hot, add the broccoli and cook for 1 minute or until bright green in color.

9. Add water and cover the skillet. Cook for 5 minutes until broccoli is tender.

10. Remove broccoli from the skillet and place in the bowl with the shrimp.

11. In a small mixing bowl, combine the remaining garlic, clam juice and cornstarch. Stir until mixture is smooth.

12. Add this mixture to the skillet and stir constantly for 5 minutes. Add in the basil, pepper, and lemon juice.

13. Return the shrimp and broccoli to the skillet and stir well. Serve.

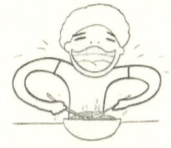

Tuna Cakes

These tuna cakes are a great play on crab cakes and taste super delicious. These cakes are only 265 calories per serving.

Ingredients:

- ¾ cup Italian seasoned breadcrumbs

- 12 ounces white tuna in water, drained and flaked

- 2 tablespoon pimentos, chopped

- ¼ cup scallions, chopped

- 1 large egg

- ½ teaspoon lemon peel, grated

- ½ cup skim milk

- 2 tablespoon butter

- 1 tablespoon lemon juice

- ¼ cup fat free chicken broth

Directions:

1. In a large mixing bowl, combine the breadcrumbs, tuna, scallions, milk, pimentos, egg, and lemon peel.

2. Lightly flour your hands and then mix together.

3. Once mixed, form into 8 patties.

4. Place butter in a large skillet and allow to melt over medium high heat.

5. Fry the tuna patties for 3 minutes on each side or until golden brown.

6. In a small saucepan, heat the broth over medium heat.

7. Stir in the lemon juice.

8. Pour the sauce over the tuna cakes.

9. Serve.

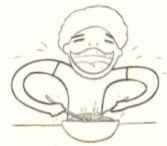

Spanish Vegetable and Pasta Bake

This is a great dinner if you are craving Spanish cuisine one night. This dinner is only 300 calories per serving and tastes great.

Ingredients:

- 2 (16 ounce) jars salsa

- 3 cups rotini pasta

- 1 (10 ounce) package frozen corn

- 1 (16 ounce) can black beans, rinsed and drained

- 2 cups shredded cheddar cheese, reduced fat

- ¼ cup cilantro, chopped

- 1 cup fat free cottage cheese

Directions:

1.	Cook the pasta according to the package
directions. Drain.

2.	In a large mixing bowl, combine the salsa, rotini,
cottage cheese, 1 cup cheddar cheese, corn and
beans. Mix well until combined.

3.	Preheat the oven to 375 degrees.

4.	Grab a 13 inch by 9 inch casserole dish and grease
with cooking spray.

5.	Spread the rotini mixture into the casserole dish.

6.	Top with remaining cheese and then place in the
oven,

7.	Bake for 25 minutes or until heated throughout.

8.	Sprinkle with cilantro and serve.

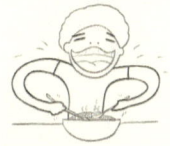

Beer Shrimp

This shrimp is delicately flavored with the beer and seasonings. You will absolutely love this way to cook shrimp and want to make it all the time. Each serving is 200 calories.

Ingredients:

- 1 tablespoon black peppercorns

- 1 tablespoon fennel seeds

- 1 teaspoon mustard seeds

- 1 tablespoon whole allspice

- 1 teaspoon whole cloves

- 1 red onion, chopped

- 2 tablespoons olive oil

- 1 garlic head, cut in half

- 2 bay leaves

- 3 jalapenos, chopped

- 3 (12 ounce) bottles light beer

- 1 tablespoon orange peel, grated

- 1 ¾ pounds shrimp

Directions:

1. Place olive oil in a skillet over medium heat.

2. Once the oil is hot, add in the peppercorns, fennel seeds, mustard seeds, cloves, and allspice. Allow to cook for 30 seconds.

3. Add in the garlic, onion, bay leaves, jalapenos, and orange peel. Stir well.

4. Reduce the heat to medium and cook for 10 minutes or until onions are tender.

5. While stirring, slowly add the beer and then allow the mixture to come to a boil.

6. Add in the shrimp and stir.

7. Cook the shrimp for 3 minutes or until they are

cooked through.

8.   Remove the shrimp from the sauce and place in a bowl.

9.   Cover the shrimp and place in the refrigerator to chill.

10. Discard the sauce and serve the shrimp cold.

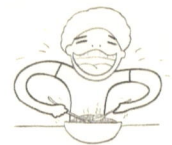

Spinach Stuffed Scallops

These scallops are stuffed with a spinach mixture that make them irresistible. You will enjoy every bite. Each serving is less than 120 calories.

Ingredients:

- 1 tablespoon cilantro, chopped

- 1 tablespoon olive oil

- 3 tablespoons spinach, chopped

- 1 tablespoon garlic, minced

- 28 sea scallops

- ½ cup white wine

- 1 tablespoon lemon juice

Directions:

1. Take each scallop and cut them in half lengthwise making sure not to cut all the way through.

2. In a mixing bowl, combine the cilantro, lemon juice, spinach, and garlic. Mix well.

3. Evenly spoon the spinach mixture into the scallops and then press the scallops to seal.

4. Heat oil in a large skillet over medium high heat.

5. Once the oil is hot, add in the scallops and brown on each side.

6. Remove the scallops from the skillet and add the white wine to the skillet.

7. Allow the wine to heat and then return the scallops to the pan and cook for an additional minute.

8. Serve.

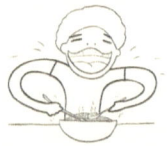

Arugula and Wild Mushroom Pizza

This is a great twist on traditional pizza and only rings in at a whopping 185 calories. Get ready to chow down!

Ingredients:

- ¼ teaspoon salt

- ¼ teaspoon pepper

- ½ pound mixed mushrooms, sliced

- 2 cups arugula leaves

- 2 tablespoon olive oil

- 1 cup grated mozzarella cheese

- Premade pizza dough

- Cornmeal for pizza dough

- 1 ½ teaspoons lemon juice

Directions:

1.   Preheat your oven to 500 degrees and sprinkle a pizza pan or stone with cornmeal.

2.   Grease a casserole dish and toss the mushrooms in 1 tablespoon of the olive oil.

3.   Season the mushrooms with salt and pepper and place in the casserole dish.

4.   Place the dish in the oven and roast the mushrooms for 10 minutes or until browned and tender.

5.   Remove the dish from the oven.

6.   In a small mixing bowl, mix the arugula, remaining olive oil, and lemon juice together. Set aside.

7.   Prepare the pizza dough in the pizza pan or on the stone and brush the outer edges with olive oil.

8.   Evenly sprinkle the cheese on top of the dough.

9.   Top with the mushrooms.

10.   Place the pizza in the oven and bake for 10 minutes or until bubbling.

11.   Remove from the oven and allow to cool slightly.

12.   Top with arugula mixture and serve.

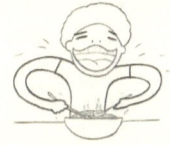

Hearty Ravioli Stew

This ravioli stew is the perfect night time meal and makes enough for a family to feast on. Each serving is under 230 calories and the flavors will pop in your mouth.

Ingredients:

- 1 onion, chopped

- 2 tablespoons olive oil

- 2 carrots, diced

- 1 red bell pepper, diced

- 2 celery ribs, diced

- 1 garlic clove, minced

- 4 plum tomatoes, chopped

- 2 ½ cups water

- 1 can (14 ounces) red kidney beans, drained and rinsed

- 1 (10 ounce) package frozen cheese ravioli, reduced fat

- 1 packet dry herb soup mix

Directions:

1. In a large saucepan over medium high heat, allow the oil to become hot.

2. Add in the onion, celery, carrots, bell pepper and garlic. Cook for 5 minutes or until tender.

3. Slowly stir in the beans, soup mix, and tomatoes. Mix well until combined.

4. Allow the mixture to come to a boil.

5. Once boiling, stir in the ravioli and then reduce the heat.

6. Cook over medium low heat for 5 minutes.

7. Serve.

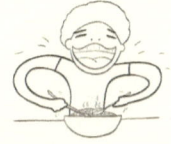

Baked Potato Soup

This soup is warming and also hearty. The potatoes are tender and come together nicely in the rich and creamy broth. Each serving is only 305 calories.

Ingredients:

- ½ cup reduced fat butter

- 6 cups skim milk

- 4 large baking potatoes

- 2 teaspoons pepper

- 2 scallions, sliced

- ½ cup flour

- 6 ounces reduced fat sour cream

- 1 onion, chopped

- 4 slices bacon, cooked and crumbled

- 1 teaspoon salt

Directions:

1. Preheat the oven to 400 degrees and wash the potatoes.

2. Once the oven is preheated, cook the potatoes for 1 hour or until tender.

3. Remove the potatoes from the oven and allow to cool.

4. Cut the potatoes in cubes.

5. In a large skillet, melt the butter over medium high heat.

6. Add in the flour and stir constantly for 1 minute.

7. Slowly whisk in the milk and continue to whisk until the mixture begins to thicken.

8. Add in the salt, potatoes, pepper, bacon, and onions. Stir well.

9. All the soup to cook for 10 minutes or until warm throughout.

10.   Add in the sour cream and stir.

11.   Serve.

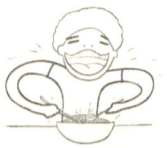

Oven Baked Crusted Catfish

This catfish is oh so tempting and delicious. The crust will be nice and crispy and the catfish extra tender and mouthwatering. This dinner is only 240 calories.

Ingredients:

- 3 ounces whole wheat crackers, crushed

- 2 pounds catfish fillets

- ¼ teaspoon salt

- 2 tablespoon butter, melted

- ¼ teaspoon hot pepper sauce

- ¾ cup reduced fat buttermilk

Directions:

1. Preheat the oven to 400 degrees and coat a baking

dish with cooking spray.

2.   In a shallow pie dish, combine the buttermilk, hot pepper sauce, and salt. Mix well.

3.   Place the crushed crackers in a separate pie dish.

4.   Take the catfish and dip it into the buttermilk mixture and then roll it in the breadcrumbs.

5.   Place the coated catfish fillets in the greased baking dish.

6.   Top the catfish fillets with the melted butter.

7.   Place in the oven and cook for 20 minutes.

8.   Remove from the oven and serve.

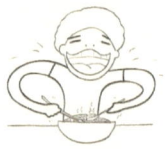

Baked Pineapple BBQ Salmon

This flaky and tender salmon is baked to perfection and dressed with a delicious barbecue sauce. Each serving of this entrée is 314 calories.

Ingredients:

- ½ teaspoon salt

- ½ teaspoon chili powder

- ½ teaspoon ground cinnamon

- 2 teaspoons lemon rind, grated

- ¼ cup pineapple juice

- 2 tablespoons light brown sugar

- 4 salmon fillets

- 2 tablespoons lemon juice

Directions:

1.   In a Ziploc bag, combine the lemon juice, salmon fillets, and pineapple juice. Toss to coat the salmon evenly and then refrigerate for 1 hour.

2.   Preheat your oven to 400 degrees and grease a 13 inch by 9 inch baking dish. Set aside.

3.   Remove the salmon from the refrigerator and the Ziploc bag.

4.   Discard the marinade and place the salmon in a shallow dish.

5.   In a small bowl, mix together the chili powder, brown sugar, salt, lemon rind, and cinnamon. Mix well and then rub over the salmon fillets to coat.

6.   Place the fish in the baking dish and place in the oven.

7.   Bake for 10-15 minutes or until fish is cooked through.

8.   Serve.

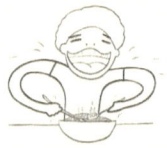

Beef and Pasta

This is a great weeknight recipe that is easy to make and can be ready in as little as 30 minutes. Each serving is only 275 calories.

Ingredients:

- ¼ cup sundried tomatoes

- 1/3 cup hot water

- 4 ounces bow tie pasta

- 1 ½ pounds boneless beef sirloin steak, sliced into 1/8 inch thick pieces

- 1 onion, chopped

- 1 pound asparagus tips

- 1 cup tomato puree

- 1 ½ cups fat free beef broth

- 2 tablespoons parmesan cheese

- 3 tablespoons basil, chopped

- ¼ teaspoon pepper

Directions:

1. Place the tomatoes in a small bowl and cover with hot water. Allow to soak for 15 minutes. Drain and chop. Set to the side.

2. Place a large skillet over medium heat and coat with cooking spray.

3. Once hot, add in the onions, asparagus and 1 cup of the beef broth.

4. Cook for 5-10 minutes or until the broth is absorbed.

5. Remove the vegetables from the skillet and set aside.

6. Add the beef to the same skillet and cook for 3 minutes or until cooked throughout.

7. Add the asparagus and onions back to the skillet and stir in the remaining beef broth.

8. Add in the remaining ingredients, except for the cheese, and stir well.

9. Cook for 15 minutes or until heated throughout.

10. Top with cheese and serve.

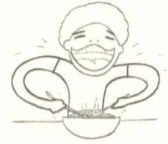

Bean Tacos

These tacos are a play on traditional tacos and made from three different beans. You will like this take on tacos and enjoy them any night of the week. Each serving carries under 150 calories.

Ingredients:

- 1 cup onion, diced

- 1 teaspoon olive oil

- ½ cup red bell pepper, diced

- ½ cup green bell pepper, diced

- 2 teaspoons dried oregano

- 1 tablespoon chili powder

- 1 garlic clove, minced

- 1 teaspoon ground cumin

- 12 taco shells

- ¾ cup tomato, diced

- ½ cup salsa

- ¾ cup iceberg lettuce, shredded

- ½ cup shredded cheddar cheese, reduced fat

- ½ cup canned black beans

- ½ cup canned pinto beans

- 1 cup canned chickpeas

Directions:

1. Drain and rinse all of the beans.

2. In a large skillet over medium high heat, allow the oil to warm.

3. Once hot, add in the onion, green pepper, red pepper, oregano, chili powder, and cumin. Mix well and allow to cook for 3 minutes.

4. Stir in the chickpeas, pinto beans, black beans, and

tomato paste.

5.   Allow the mixture to reach a boil and then reduce the heat.

6.   Simmer for 20 minutes or until the sauce is thickened.

7.   Get the taco shells ready according to the package directions.

8.   Spoon ¼ cup of the bean mixture into each of the taco shells.

9.   Top each taco with cheese, tomato, lettuce and salsa.

10.   Serve.

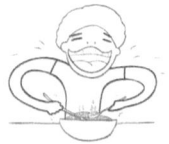

Delicious Pierogi and Chicken Soup

This soup is nicely flavored with the chicken and cheese Pierogies. Each serving is less than 300 calories. This dish will warm you from the inside out with every bite.

Ingredients:

- 1 ½ pounds boneless, skinless chicken breasts, cut into bite sized pieces

- 28 mini frozen cheese pierogies

- 1 tablespoon vegetable oil

- ¼ cup flour

- ¼ cup onion, minced

- ½ teaspoon minced garlic

- 1/8 teaspoon nutmeg

- 2 cups skim milk

- 3 cups spinach, chopped

- 1 (14 ounce) can chicken broth, fat free

- ¼ teaspoon pepper

- ¼ teaspoon salt

Directions:

1. Place the pierogies in a saucepan of boiling water and cook for 3 minutes or until thawed.

2. Drain and place in a bowl. Set to the side.

3. In a large Dutch oven, heat oil over medium high heat.

4. Once oil is hot, add in the chicken, garlic and onion. Stir and cook for 5 minutes or until chicken is lightly golden brown.

5. Add in the flour and continue to stir for 1 minute.

6. Slowly stir in the rest of the ingredients and allow the mixture to come to a boil.

7. Reduce the heat and let simmer for 10 minutes.

8.   Add in the pierogies and cook for an additional 5 minutes.

9.   Serve.

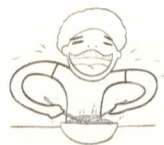

Superlicious Spinach and Mushroom Quiche

This quiche is made with mushrooms and is very tasty and satisfying. You can eat this quiche for dinner and enjoy it whenever you want. Each serving is under 120 calories.

Ingredients:

- 1 onion, chopped

- 2 cups mushrooms, sliced

- ¼ cup plain breadcrumbs

- 1 (10 ounce) package frozen spinach, thawed and drained

- 2 cups skim milk

- 1 teaspoon garlic powder

- ½ teaspoon pepper

- 1 teaspoon Italian seasoning

- ¼ cup parmesan cheese

- 8 large egg whites

Directions:

1. Preheat your oven to 350 degrees and grease a quiche pan with cooking spray.

2. In a skillet over medium high heat, saute the mushrooms and onions for 5 minutes or until tender.

3. Add in the spinach and continue to cook for an additional 5 minutes.

4. Stir in the breadcrumbs.

5. Pour the mixture into your greased quiche pan.

6. Place all of the remaining ingredients in a separate bowl and mix together.

7. Pour over the spinach mixture evenly.

8.   Place in the oven and bake for 40 minutes or until
        the eggs are set.

9.   Remove from the oven and allow to cool slightly
        before slicing.

10.   Serve.

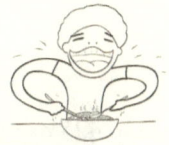

Vegetable Calzones

These calzones are a great way to get your calzone fix without all of the carbs and calories in a real calzone. The vegetables in this calzone are tender yet crispy enough for you to enjoy and the meal come in at 250 calories.

Ingredients:

- 1 large egg white, scrambled

- ¾ cup mushrooms, sliced

- ½ cup red bell pepper, diced

- ¾ cup zucchini, sliced thin

- ¼ teaspoon dried basil

- 1 (10 ounce) can refrigerated pizza crust

- ¼ teaspoon garlic salt

- 1 cup shredded mozzarella cheese, reduced fat

- ¼ cup scallions, diced

Directions:

1. Preheat your oven to 425 degrees and grease a baking sheet with cooking spray.

2. In a large mixing bowl, combine the zucchini, onion, pepper, and mushrooms. Add in the basil and garlic salt. Toss well.

3. Unroll the pizza dough and shape into a 14 inch square pizza.

4. Cut the dough into 4 equal pieces.

5. Sprinkle ¼ cup of the cheese onto each of the 4 slices of dough.

6. Top each piece of dough with ¼ of the vegetable mixture.

7. Fold the dough in half and seal the edges to keep the mixture in.

8. Place the calzones on the baking sheet and brush with the egg white.

9. Bake in the oven for 15 minutes or until done and golden brown.

10. Serve.

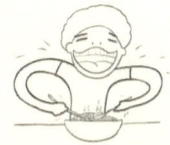

Chicken Soup with Wild Rice

This soup is the perfect blend of rice and chicken. It is hearty and also very filling. You can even eat leftovers for lunch the next day. Each servings has under 250 calories.

Ingredients:

- 2 (14 ounce) cans chicken broth, fat free

- 1 package (6 ounces) wild rice mix

- 4 garlic cloves, minced

- ¼ teaspoon pepper

- 4 cups tomatoes, chopped

- 1 tablespoon thyme

- 1 cup zucchini, diced

- 1 (9 ounce) package of frozen chicken breast, chopped

- 1 tablespoon dry sherry

Directions:

1. Prepare the rice on the stove according to the directions on the package. Once the rice is done cooking, do not add in any butter or seasonings. Set aside.

2. In a large Dutch oven, combine the thyme, chicken broth, and garlic. Allow the mixture to come to a boil.

3. Stir in the zucchini, tomatoes, chicken, and pepper.

4. Allow the mixture to return to a boil and then reduce the heat.

5. Cover the pot and allow to simmer for 5 minutes.

6. Stir in the rice and wine. Continue heating for 5 minutes.

7. Serve.

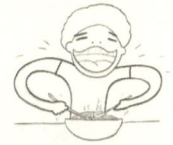

Easy Vegetable Stroganoff

This is a different take on traditional beef stroganoff and you will love the blend of noodles with the tender vegetables. Cooking this in the slow cooker really does make a difference. Each serving is under 330 calories.

Ingredients:

- ½ cup onion, diced

- 1 teaspoon olive oil

- 1 ¼ cup frozen broccoli

- 1 tablespoon minced garlic

- 3 cups mushrooms, sliced

- 2 carrots, chopped

- 1 cup vegetable broth

- 2 tablespoons tomato paste

- 4 cups egg noodles, cooked

- ¼ cup fat free yogurt, plain

- ¼ cup reduced fat sour cream

- 2 teaspoons cornstarch

Directions:

1. Heat oil in a skillet over medium heat.

2. Add the onion and saute for 5 minutes or until tender.

3. Add in the garlic and mushrooms. Continue cooking for another 5 minutes.

4. Add this mixture to your slow cooker.

5. Add the carrots, broccoli, vegetable broth, and tomato paste to the slow cooker as well.

6. Stir the mixture well and then cover.

7. Cook on medium for 4 hours or until most of the liquid has been absorbed.

8. In a small saucepan, combine the sour cream, cornstarch, and yogurt.

9. Allow to warm on the stove until heated through.

10. Pour the sauce over the vegetables and stir well.

11. Serve over the egg noodles.

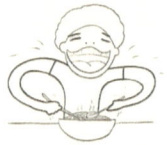

Hashbrown, Veggie, and Cheese Bake

This delicious bake is easy to make and is delicious above all. The hashbrowns keep you coming back for another bite again and again. Each serving is only 200 calories.

Ingredients:

- 1 cup shredded cheddar cheese, reduced fat

- 4 ½ cups frozen shredded hashbrowns

- ¾ cup egg substitute

- ¼ teaspoon pepper

- ½ teaspoon salt

- ¼ cup tomato, chopped

- ¾ cup skim milk

- ¼ cup red bell pepper, chopped

- 3 tablespoons onion, chopped

Directions:

1. Preheat your oven to 350 degrees and grease a 9 inch pie plate with cooking spray.

2. In a large mixing bowl, combine all of the ingredients and then pour into the pie plate.

3. Bake in the oven for 45 minutes or until cooked throughout the center.

4. Serve.

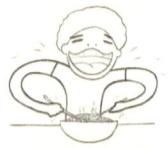

Vegetable Pizza

This pizza is packed full of tasty vegetable flavors. You will love the earthy yet cheesy taste of this pizza that is only 332 calories per serving.

Ingredients:

- 2 garlic cloves, minced

- ½ cup onion, chopped

- 1 tablespoon plus 2 teaspoons olive oil

- 1 cup eggplant, peeled and chopped

- 4 tomatoes, chopped

- 1 tablespoon thyme

- ¼ teaspoon salt

- ½ teaspoon sugar

- 1/8 teaspoon pepper

- 2 yellow tomatoes, halved

- 2 tablespoons olives, chopped

- 1 yellow summer squash, sliced

- 1 zucchini, sliced

- ½ cup shredded mozzarella cheese, reduced fat

- 16 ounces Italian bread shell

Directions:

1. Heat a skillet over medium heat and add in 2 teaspoons of olive oil.

2. Once oil is hot, add in the garlic and onion. Cook for 5 minutes or until tender.

3. Add in the eggplant, tomatoes, thyme, salt, pepper, and sugar. Cook for 15 minutes or until no more liquid remains in the pan.

4. Preheat the oven to 400 degrees and grease a baking sheet.

5. Place the bread shell on the baking sheet and layer

the skillet mixture on top of the bread shell.

6. Arrange the halved tomatoes, squash, and zucchini on top.

7. Drizzle with the remaining olive oil and sprinkle with olives and feta cheese.

8. Top with the mozzarella cheese.

9. Bake in the oven for 15 minutes or until cheese is melted and vegetables are heated.

10. Serve.

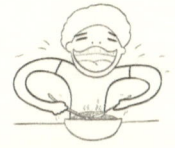

Delicious Fish
with a Black Bean Side

This recipe is perfect if you love fish and also black beans. The black bean mash is very flavorful. This recipe is easy to make and will delight. This recipe is only 200 calories.

Ingredients:

- 4 teaspoons olive oil

- 3 garlic cloves, minced

- 6 cod fillets

- 2 tablespoons lime juice

- 1 (14 ounce) can diced tomatoes

- 1 teaspoon ground cumin

- 1 (4 ounce) can diced green chilies

- ¼ teaspoon salt

- ¼ teaspoon pepper

- 1 onion, diced

- 1 (15 ounce) can black beans, drained and rinsed

Directions:

1. Rinse off the cod fillets and then dry them by patting with a paper towel. Place a large skillet over medium high heat.

2. Using 2 teaspoons of oil, brush both sides of the cod fillets.

3. Cook the fillets in the skillet for 3 minutes or until browned on the one side.

4. Flip over the fillets and cover the skillet. Reduce the heat to medium and allow to cook for 5 more minutes.

5. Remove the fish from the skillet and set aside.

6. Add the remaining oil to the skillet and allow to heat.

7. Once hot, add in the garlic and onion. Cook for 5

minutes.

8.   Season with the cumin and cook an additional minute.

9.   Add in the chilies, tomatoes, and beans. Stir well.

10. Cover and allow to cook over low heat for an additional ten minutes.

11. Stir in the salt, pepper, and lime juice.

12. Serve with the fish.

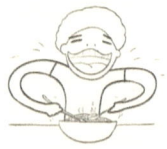

Citrus Shrimp and Asparagus

This delicious dinner is under 300 calories and is perfect for any seafood and vegetable lover. The shrimp is flavored with a nice hint of citrus flavor which will keep you craving more.

Ingredients:

- 1 cup couscous

- 2 cups water

- ½ teaspoon black pepper

- ½ teaspoon salt

- 1 tablespoon lime juice

- 4 tablespoons lemon juice

- 2 garlic cloves, minced

- 3 ½ tablespoon olive oil

- ¾ pound large shrimp, deveined and peeled

- 1 teaspoon honey

- ¾ pound asparagus spears, trimmed

- ¼ cup chives

Directions:

1. Place the 2 cups of water in a saucepan and allow to come to a boil over high heat.

2. Remove the pan from the heat and stir in the couscous. Cover and allow to sit for 5 minutes.

3. Remove the cover and stir in ¼ teaspoon salt, ¼ teaspoon pepper, and 1 tablespoon of the lemon juice. Set aside.

4. Grab another saucepan and allow it to come to a boil over high heat.

5. In a small bowl, mix together 1 tablespoon lemon juice, 1 tablespoon lime juice, garlic, salt, pepper, and 1 ½ teaspoons olive oil.

6. Add shrimp and toss. Allow to marinate for 5 minutes.

7. Preheat your grill at this point and coat the grill with cooking spray.

8. Place the shrimp on the grill and grill for 5 minutes or until cooked through.

9. Remove from the grill and bring inside.

10. Add the asparagus to the boiling pot of water and cook for 4 minutes or until tender. Drain.

11. In a small bowl, whisk together the chives, honey, remaining olive oil, and remaining lemon juice.

12. Place the couscous and asparagus on a plate. Top with the shrimp and drizzle the dressing on top. Serve.

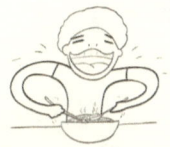

Teriyaki Chicken with Noodles

This is the perfect Chinese at home take out dinner. Under 350 calories, this dish is so delicious you will want to eat it again and again.

Ingredients:

- 5 ounces soba noodles, uncooked

- 1 pound boneless, skinless chicken breasts

- 2 cups low sodium chicken broth

- ¼ cup plus 1 ½ tablespoons teriyaki sauce

- 2 teaspoons ginger, peeled and grated

- 2 cups water

- 7 ounces mushrooms, sliced

- 2 garlic cloves, minced

- 3 carrots, grated

- 2 teaspoons sesame oil

- 4 scallions, sliced

- ¼ cup cilantro, chopped

- ¼ cup basil, chopped

- 4 radishes, sliced

Directions:

1. Place the chicken and ¼ cup of the teriyaki sauce in a bowl and allow to marinate for 30 minutes.

2. Preheat a grill and coat with cooking spray.

3. Grill the chicken for 15 minutes or until cooked through.

4. Remove from the grill and wrap in aluminum foil.

5. In a saucepan, combine the water, chicken broth, garlic, ginger, and teriyaki sauce until well combined.

6. Allow the mixture to come to a boil.

7. Add in the scallions, mushrooms, and carrots. Reduce heat and simmer for 10 minutes.

8.   Boil the soba noodles in a separate saucepan for 5 minutes or until tender. Drain and divide equally into serving bowls.

9.   Add the sesame oil, cilantro and bail to the simmering broth. Stir and then divide evenly into the bowls.

10.   Slice the wrapped chicken and add to the bowls.

11.   Serve.

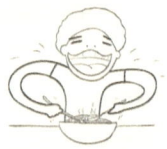

Crispy Chicken Nuggets with Blackberry Sauce

These chicken nuggets are only 185 calories per serving and are nice and crispy. They go great with the delicious blackberry jam served with them. Enjoy these any day of the week for dinner.

Ingredients:

- 1 ½ tablespoons mustard

- 1 cup fresh blackberries, minced

- 1 pound chicken tender, cut in half

- 2 teaspoons honey

- 3 tablespoons cornmeal

- ¼ teaspoon pepper

- 1 tablespoon olive oil

- ½ teaspoon salt

Directions:

1. In a small bowl, mash the blackberries until all are mashed.

2. Add in the honey and mustard and mix well. Set aside.

3. Season the chicken with salt and pepper.

4. Place the cornmeal in a shallow pie dish and dip each chicken tender in the cornmeal. Coat evenly.

5. Place oil in a skillet and allow to heat over medium high heat.

6. Cook the chicken in the skillet for 10 minutes or until done in the center.

7. Serve the nuggets on a plate with some of the blackberry sauce.

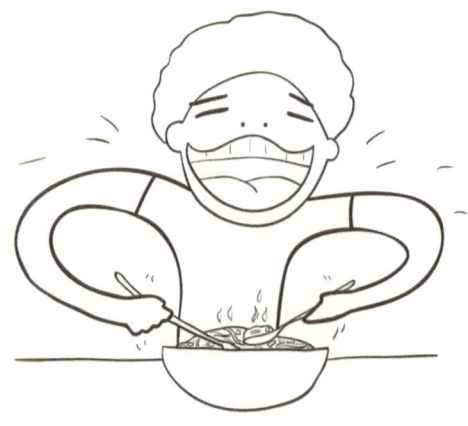

A Final Word of Encouragement

Thank you so much for reading!

If, like so many, you have tried again and again to lose weight with this or that diet trend, let me encourage you right now. The Fast Diet has worked really well for lots of people. We realize that we have not given you an encyclopedia of Fast Diet recipes – instead we have chosen a really useful range of real meals that will work for you on a day to day basis to get the kind of results you are looking to achieve.

Keep those lips smackin' and enjoy every awesome morsel.